Treat Arthritis The Natural Way

Your Arthritis Handbook to Natural Pain Relief

Ron Kness

Treat Arthritis The Natural Way Contents

Published by:

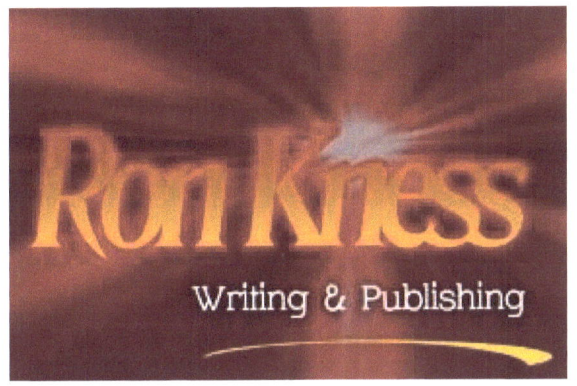

https://ronknesswriting.com

Ron Kness

San Tan Valley, AZ

United States of America

ISBN: 9781091442542

Introduction

Arthritis is a condition which adversely affects the lifestyles of many ... me for one. It causes discomfort, pain and decreased mobility. Although it is widespread, arthritis, and its causes and effects, are often greatly misunderstood.

Many think that arthritis is one simple condition, not realizing that that there are dozens of distinct conditions that are classified as arthritis, some with very different symptoms, treatments and how the condition is contracted in the first place.

Probably the single most common factor in all, is the pain and lessened mobility, greatly due in part to the pain.

For sufferers, the greatest knowledge that they may be unaware of is that in most cases the symptoms do not have to be considered inevitable, to be borne for the rest of their life.

Research and data-sharing has proven that for many suffering from different types of arthritis, the symptoms and degree of pain can be reduced, and range of movement increased, by changes in diet and lifestyle.

Pharmaceutical treatments exist, and many have become dependent on them, however effective, natural options are available and have helped many to reduce the incidence and effects of their condition. In some cases, the side effects from the pharmaceutical treatment is worse than what it is trying to treat. To prove that point, read my story in the Conclusion of this book.

Those who don't (yet) suffer from arthritis may better understand how changes to their lifestyle, especially diet, can help reduce their likelihood of being affected by arthritis in their future.

Common Arthritis Types

The word "Arthritis" originates from "arthro," which translates to "joint," and "itis," which translates to "inflammation." Amazingly, this term is used to comprise over 100 different, yet related conditions.

For example, these joint issues can range from relatively mild cases of bursitis or tendonitis to much more severe and crippling forms of inflammation, such as rheumatoid arthritis and osteoarthritis – the latter of which I have.

Conditions known as pain syndromes, such as fibromyalgia, as well as systemic lupus erythematous which involves every portion of the body, are also related. Other representations of the disease, such as gout, are additionally related, however, they are rarely connected.

Pain in The Joints

The common thread connecting the above-mentioned diseases is musculoskeletal pain and joint pain. This is why these varied conditions are grouped together under the common umbrella called "arthritis."

Inflammation is often the body's natural response to injury, and inflammation of the lining within the joints is common.

Additional symptoms include pain, the affected joint being hot to the touch, swelling and redness. Once the joint is inflamed, it may develop all of these symptoms or a portion of them. Obviously, this can become excruciating and the normal movement of the joint can become extremely limited. Everyday activities may become difficult and loss of motion can occur.

Different Types of Arthritis

Unfortunately, arthritis can affect anyone, although some specific types affect certain demographics more. There are several types of arthritis that may affect people of any age, race or gender.

Fortunately, there are steps that can be taken to help the body facilitate healing and help to eliminate or reduce the inflammatory response that is responsible for the condition.

Arthritis at Any Age

Children and babies as well as young adults can suffer from this condition. Statistics show that approximately 3 people out of 5 who have arthritis are under 65 years of age.

Rheumatoid Arthritis

Rheumatoid arthritis is the type of arthritis that can cause the bones to appear disfigured or deformed. It's an insidious disease whereby the body's own immune system attacks the joints and surrounding tissues, and in some cases cause problems in other parts of the body.

It causes painful swelling, in which case anti-inflammatory medications are prescribed as there is no natural cure.

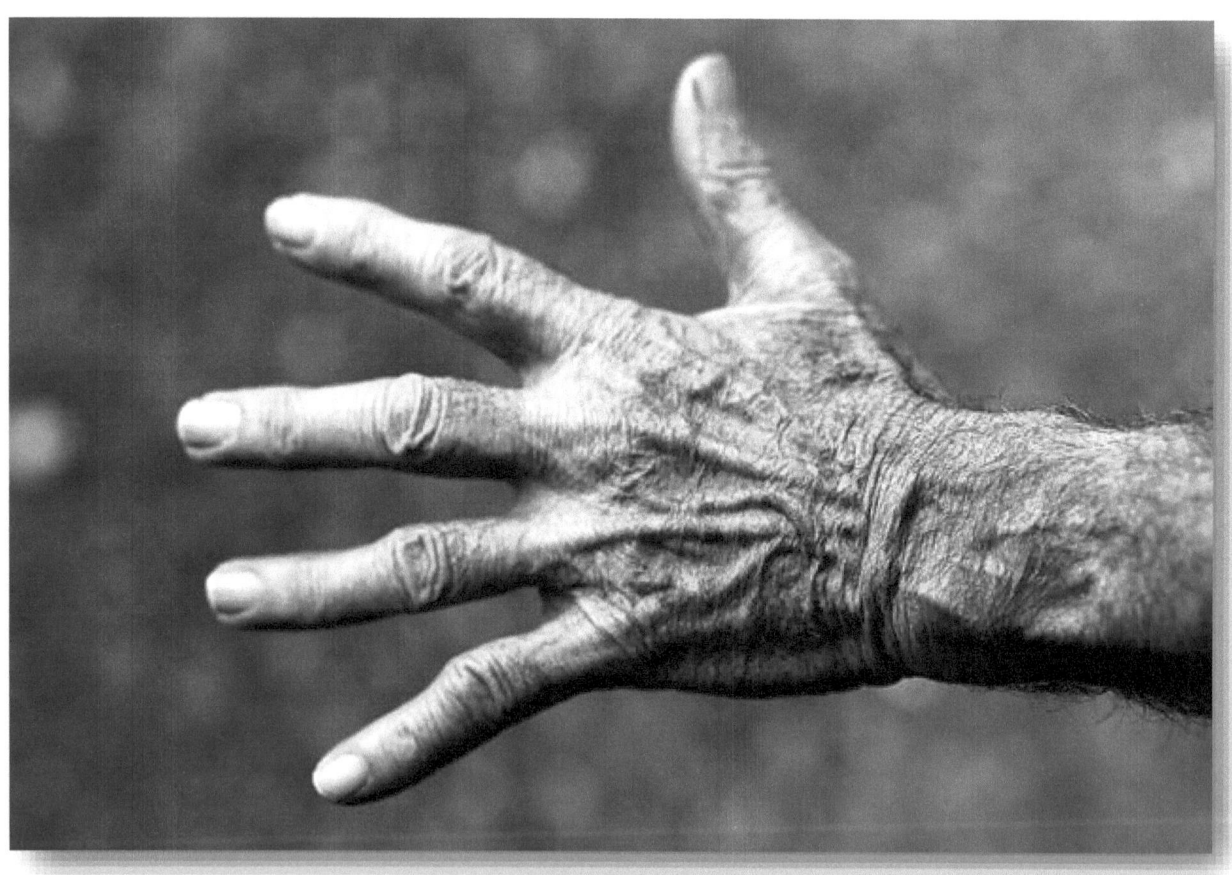

Juvenile Rheumatoid Arthritis

This condition is also called idiopathic arthritis. This type of arthritis affects children and adolescents below the age of sixteen. Reddish, swollen joints accompanied by pain are some of the most common symptoms.

Some children and adolescents experience its symptoms for just a few months, while others suffer for the rest of their lives. Treatment is mostly focused on keeping the pain under control, preventing the occurrence of any complications and in improving the mobility and joint functions.

Osteoarthritis

Often called "wear and tear arthritis." This type is characterized by stiffness and joint pain due to cartilage erosion within in a joint. It commonly affects the hips, hands, spine and knees in menopausal women and the elderly.

Psoriatic Arthritis

Fingers and toes are the areas' most susceptible to this kind of joint erosion arthritis that affects patients with psoriasis. Fingernails may become deeply ridged and pitted in affected individuals.

Gout or Gouty Arthritis

This acute form of arthritis results from a disturbance of protein metabolism in the body. In this situation, uric acid production is increased and deposits of uric acid crystals can accumulate within the joints. The toes, fingers and knees are most commonly affected.

Normally, excess crystals are eliminated via the urine. However, they can build up and cause crystal formation if any issues arise with the elimination process. If left untreated, the arterial system can become affected.

An individual with this type of arthritis will experience sudden attacks of joint pain accompanied by redness and swelling in the affected area.

In most cases, the joint on the big toe is the first one to be affected while the toes on the other side of the body as well as the knees can also experience pain.

Men are ten times more likely to suffer from this condition than women. People who are obese, overweight, alcoholic (or drink in excess), face a higher risk of having gouty arthritis.

Pseudogout Arthritis

This type of arthritis commonly affects the wrists and knees. However, it may also affect the ankles, finger joints, shoulders, hips and elbows. Pseudoarthritis occurs when the calcium pyrophosphate crystals (CPP) accumulate in the cartilage.

The formation of CPP can be caused by having abnormal cells in the cartilage. It can also be caused by injury and/or surgery. In some cases, pseudogout arthritis can also be hereditary.

Infectious Arthritis

This form of arthritis results from an infection caused by bacteria, fungi or a virus that gets into the bloodstream affecting the joints. It can also occur as a result of an infection in an area near the joint. Infectious arthritis can either be acute or chronic.

- *Chronic infectious arthritis* is caused by fungi, or mycobacterium that also causes tuberculosis. This type of infectious arthritis develops gradually over a period of several weeks.

- *Acute infectious arthritis* can be caused by viruses and bacteria. This type of arthritis can develop quickly and the cartilage or joint affected can be damaged within a few hours or days.

Hemorrhagic Arthritis

This type of arthritis results from the blood getting into the person's joints leading to inflammation, and may occur as a result of trauma, injury, lesion or cut to the joint. People who have hemophilia A, hemophilia B and sickle cell disease face a higher risk of hemorrhagic arthritis.

Therapy for this kind of arthritis will usually depend on its cause.

There are many types of arthritis, so don't self-diagnose. If you feel any pain in the joints, check with your health care professional.

Rheumatoid Arthritis

Rheumatoid arthritis causes joint pain and is a systemic disease, meaning it spreads throughout the body. It is also an auto-immune disease. This is when your body's immune system which normally protects you against disease causing bacteria and viruses, mistakenly attacks your joints.

When your autoimmune system attacks the thin membrane that lines your joints, systemic inflammation and pain will start to occur. This systemic inflammation can also lead to a loss of appetite and fatigue and decline in overall health. Muscle wasting and anemia may also occur.

However, with early diagnosis and correct treatment, you can prevent rheumatoid arthritis from causing further damage to your joints, ligaments, cartilage and tendons. It commonly affects fingers, wrists and elbows.

Rheumatoid arthritis is a symmetrical condition and typically, the erosive changes develop on a symmetrical basis This means that if your joint on the left side of your body is affected, the other corresponding joint on the right side of your body will also be affected.

Inflammation may cause the synovial membrane between the joints to thicken and eventually, cartilage wears away and the bony fusion can lead to a joint becoming permanently fixated.

What Are the Symptoms of Rheumatoid Arthritis?

The severity of the condition may vary from one person to another. Many sufferers with this condition will say they experience intermittent bouts of pain or 'flare-ups' which can become worse over a period of time. These flares may last for one day or for several months.

The most common symptoms include reddish, swollen, warm joints. Often there is joint stiffness, which usually occurs in the morning, with the pain lessening in intensity during the day.

If you experience a recurring and unexplained tingling feeling or numbness in your hands and wrists or pain in your fore-foot, you may be suffering from rheumatoid arthritis.

Other not so common symptoms may include dryness of the mouth, eyes, throat, skin and nose. This is due to the autoimmune disorder that causes certain glands to stop releasing moisture. This dryness in several parts of the body can be experienced even when rheumatoid arthritis is still in its early stages.

What Are the Causes of Rheumatoid Arthritis?

Today, the exact causes have not yet been fully understood. If some members of your family have the condition, the likelihood of you developing the condition is a higher risk probability.

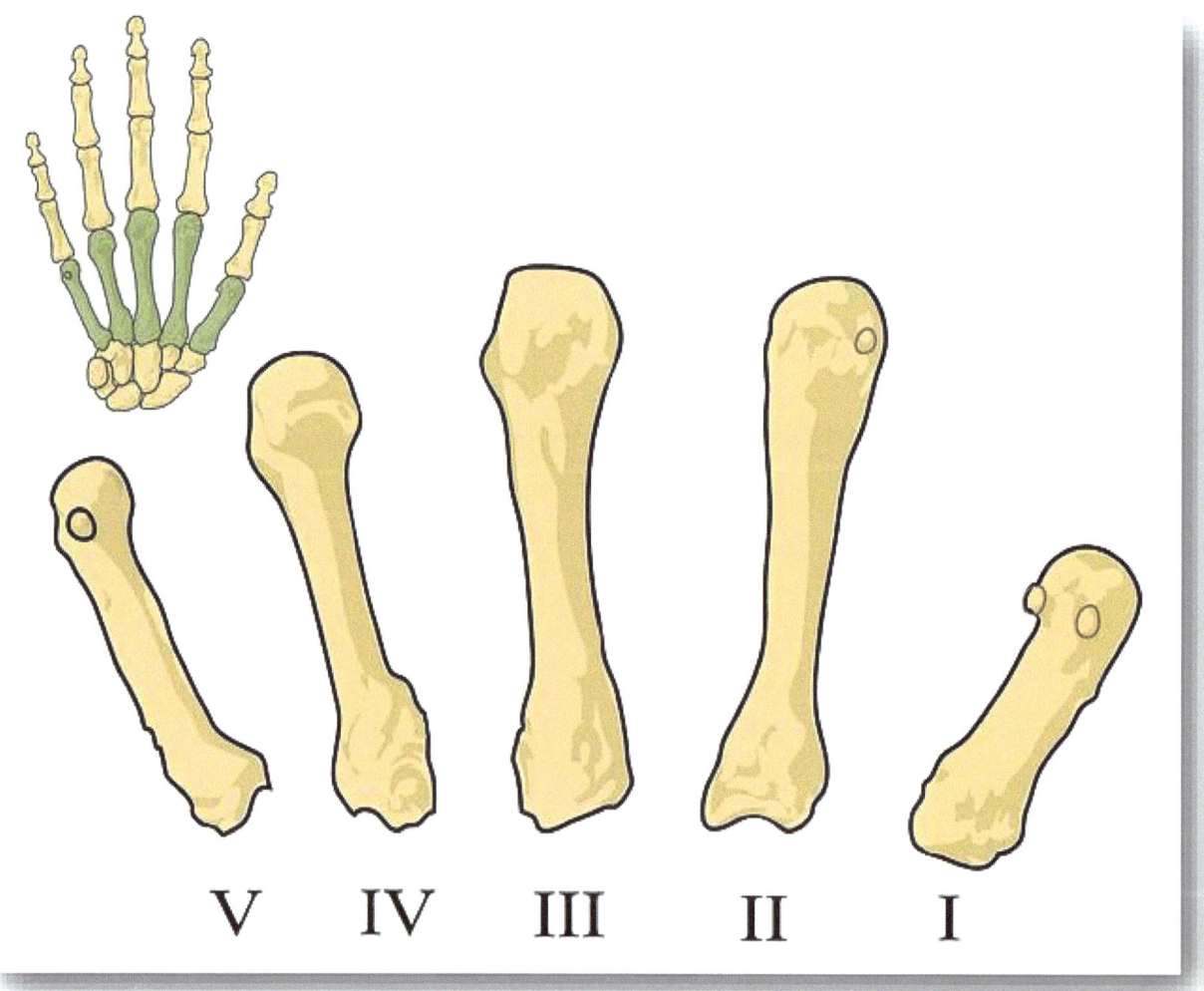

Several lifestyle factors may also come into play in increasing your risks of developing rheumatoid arthritis. For example, smoking, hormonal changes and stress have been causally linked to the condition.

What Are the Long-Term Side Effects?

One of the most common long term side effects is limited movement and joint deformity. Lumps of tissue called 'rheumatoid nodules' may also develop under the skin where the bones are located.

The internal systems and organs of the body can also be affected due to the condition causing systemic or body-wide inflammation.

Unfortunately, since a cure for this condition has not yet been discovered, those who have been diagnosed with this disease may suffer from it chronically for life.

Prevention

Preventive measures include Vitamin C, as synovia or joint fluids seem to be the object of attack. The vitamin C is an antioxidant and helps to build collagen and fight the inflammation.

Osteoarthritis

Osteoarthritis is the most common type of arthritis. It is also referred to as the "wear and tear" arthritis or degenerative joint disease. This condition occurs when the cartilage wears away. The cartilage functions as a buffer and helps cushion the movement between the surfaces of the joints. If the cartilage starts to break down due to heavy use or age, osteoarthritis can start to develop.

This type of arthritis usually occurs in weight-bearing joints such as the knees, spine and hips. It can also be present in the large toes, neck, fingers and thumb.

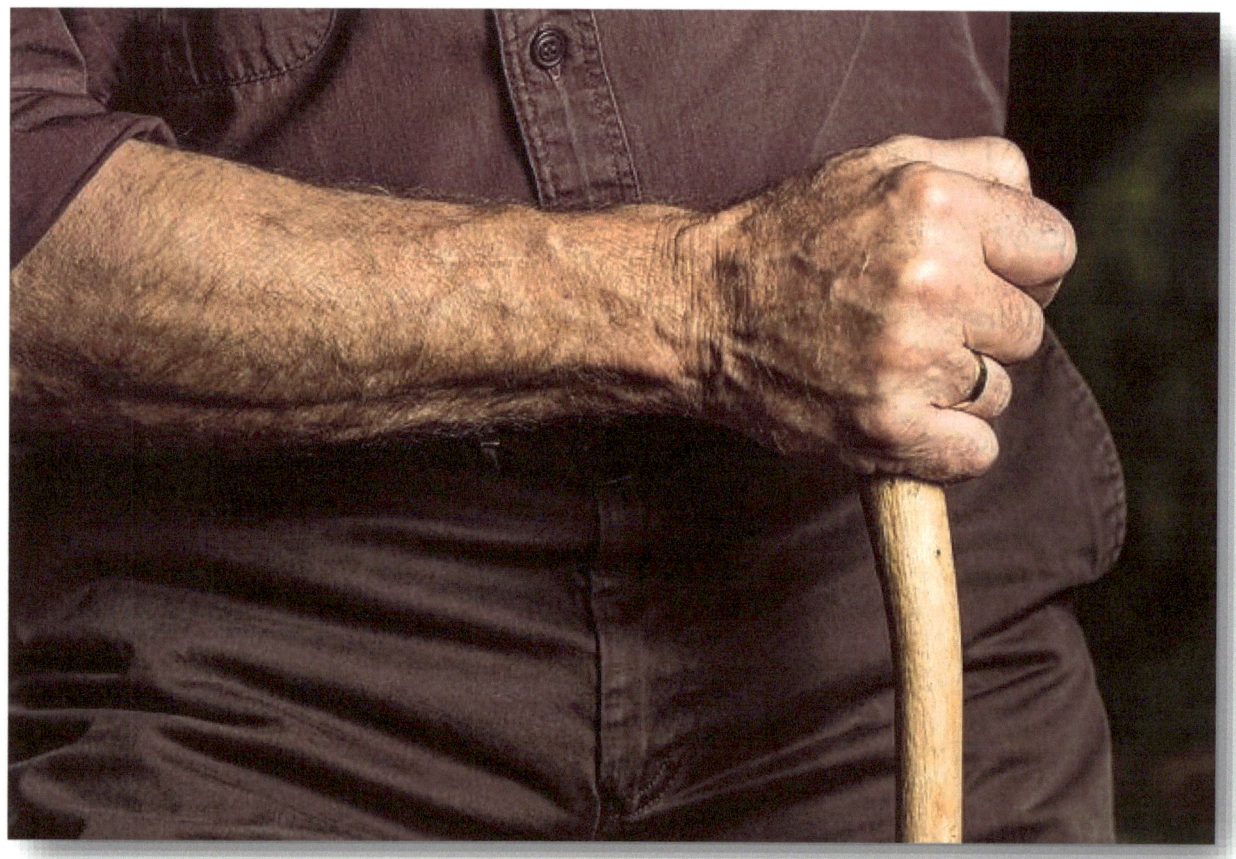

Osteoarthritis is NOT a Systemic Disease

Unlike rheumatoid arthritis, which is a systemic disease, osteoarthritis is a localized disease. Most cases of osteoarthritis are only limited to the affected area of the joints.

However, when there is a severe loss of cartilage the person may expect misshapen joints and this results in joint instability. This joint instability can also cause the joints to buckle or lock, which usually occurs in the knees.

Symptoms of Osteoarthritis

The symptoms are usually felt in the affected areas such as the knees, hips, spine, fingers and hands. Those who have osteoarthritis will most likely experience the following discomforts:

Pain

The primary symptom of osteoarthritis is pain which is also the main cause of functional impairment. Although the pain may develop gradually, it can also worsen with too much physical activity. During the early stages of OA, the pain may be reduced after resting.

Unfortunately, as the disease progresses, the pain will become more persistent making it harder for the person to experience relief, even after resting or using any type of treatment.

Joint Stiffness

Any feelings of joint stiffness can be worse in the morning. It can also be experienced after long periods of rest or inactivity. When stiffness occurs, the joints become rigid, painful and hard to move. This is why an individual's coordination, ability to observe proper posture and the ability to move freely can be affected.

Tenderness

Tenderness is a symptom that is more common to people who are already suffering the advanced stages of osteoarthritis. Tenderness can be felt when light pressure is applied to the affected joints.

Swelling

Although swelling is a more common symptom of people who have rheumatoid arthritis, it can also be experienced by people with osteoarthritis. As the cartilage wears away, bone-on-bone contact can occur and this can then lead to swelling.

Bone Spurs

Bone spurs are small bony projections. Although these bony projections may occur naturally, they can occur as a result of an inflammation to some parts of the joints. They can be painful, especially when they are rubbed against bones and/or nerves. These bone spurs are often described by osteoarthritis sufferers as hard little lumps that are felt around the affected joints.

Noisy Joints

Noisy joints are sometimes called 'crepitus' and this is common among osteoarthritis sufferers. The sound is described as being something that is grinding, crackling, creaking or snapping.

Treatment for Osteoarthritis

There is no cure for osteoarthritis but there are plenty of treatments available that will help relieve the pain. Some doctors advise osteoarthritis sufferers to undergo therapy from a professional physical therapist or occupational therapist. This type of treatment helps the person to improve their mobility.

Increasing Your Body's Flexibility

This is one part of the treatment plan that many people tend to overlook, mainly because movement is painful.

Consider taking up Yoga or Pilates to boost the flexibility of your joints and improve the strength of your muscles. When your muscles are strengthened, there will also be lesser pressure on your cartilage.

Diet and exercise are crucial to the health of the joints and bones and important for improving the body's flexibility. Increased flexibility in the joints means improved nourishment in the cartilage.

Know the Activities to Avoid

If you think that a certain activity will only cause you a lot of pain, find a better way to accomplish the task. You can make compromises to help protect your affected joints. If a task requires you to normally stand but it can be performed while sitting, do it. Try not to put too much pressure on your joints.

You also need to avoid tasks that require heavy lifting. Your common sense will tell you which tasks will be harmful, so be prepared to make some changes, or have someone else do it for you instead.

Make Use of Supportive Devices

Osteoarthritis patients may find using supportive devices to reduce the stress on their affected joints beneficial. Supportive devices have been proven helpful in stabilizing damaged joints.

Be wary of becoming reliant on any type of supportive devices, as over-use may lead to muscle wasting. Therefore, make sure to only use these devices under the supervision or advice of your doctor or therapist. There are braces, crutches, canes, shoe lifts and inserts that are helpful for reducing the pressure on the affected joints while your body and mobility improve.

Regular exercise and maintaining a healthy weight are critical, not just in terms of managing the condition, but also in slowing down its progression.

If the disease continues to become worse, surgery has been recommended as a last resort. Many osteoarthritis patients have been able to live an active life after having a joint replacement.

Gout

Gout or gouty arthritis is common among older individuals, especially men more than women. It is mainly due to the accumulation of uric acid crystal deposits in the joints.

This type of arthritis occurs when the levels of uric acid in the body is persistently very high, and uric acid crystals form in the joints and cause almost unbearable pain.

Gout is diagnosed through a blood test where the amount of uric acid in the blood is measured. An x-ray can be performed to determine the severity of the gout to the joints.

What Causes Gout?

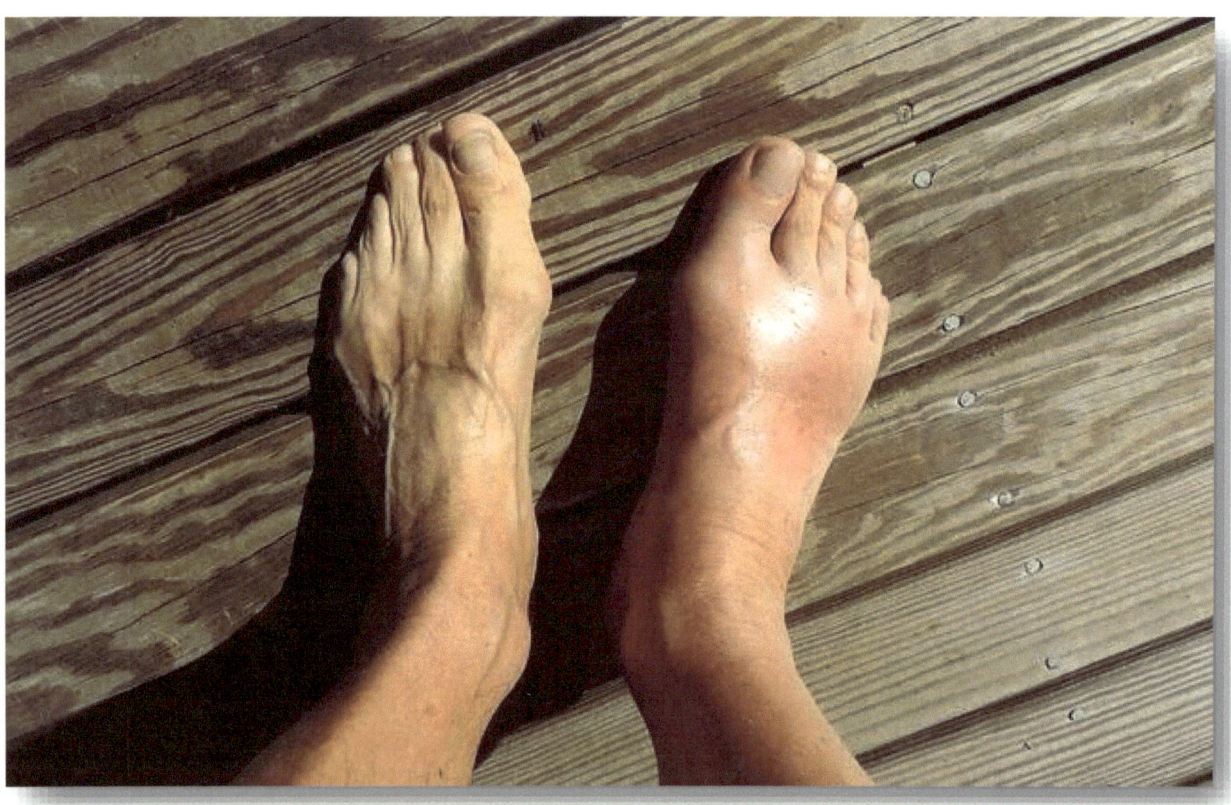

Gout usually develops due to lifestyle and diet. This condition can be caused by over indulging in purine-rich foods, such as eating high volumes of organ meats and other meats, including pork, bacon, beef and lamb, and drinking too much beer. Other alcohol consumption, obesity, and old age can also contribute to gout.

What Are the Symptoms?

Gout attacks usually occur at night or early morning. There is a significant visible swelling and redness of the joints, a sense of tenderness, and a sharp pain in the affected areas.

The most common signs of gout are pain, swelling, tenderness and redness in the smaller joints of the extremities. Gout will first attack the joints of the toes and fingers and will work its way up to the wrists, ankles, knees, etc.

Gouty arthritis can take months or years to develop, and isn't relieved easily. It can hasten the deterioration of joints.

Traditional Treatments for Gout

Medical practitioners may prescribe corticosteroids to relieve the pain of a gout attack. Anti-inflammatory medications like ibuprofen are also prescribed to alleviate the acute pain and inflammation.

Aspirin shouldn't be taken at all, as it tends to increase the blood uric acid levels.

Medications to lower uric acid levels are also prescribed, but the main disadvantages of uric acid medications is their side effects. Prolonged intake of medications can be detrimental to the body, especially the kidneys and liver.

Natural Treatments for Gout

Instead of managing uric acid levels with medications, you can choose a diet and lifestyle to prevent and manage the problem. Here are a few natural treatments listed below.

Diet

Avoid eating purine-rich foods as mentioned earlier. Fatty meats and alcoholic beverages are your main enemies. They contribute to your uric acid accumulation, so eliminate or reduce them as much as possible.

Instead add foods rich in potassium and vitamin C, such as bananas and citrus fruits, to help relieve inflammation. Potassium and vitamin C lowers uric acid levels and helps prevent inflammation and pain during gout attacks.

Eat raw fruits and vegetables as they have a neutralizing effect against uric acid. When experiencing a gout attack, some people find eating a handful of cherries or a bowl of green vegetables helpful in relieving pain.

Keep Hydrated – Drink Lots of Water

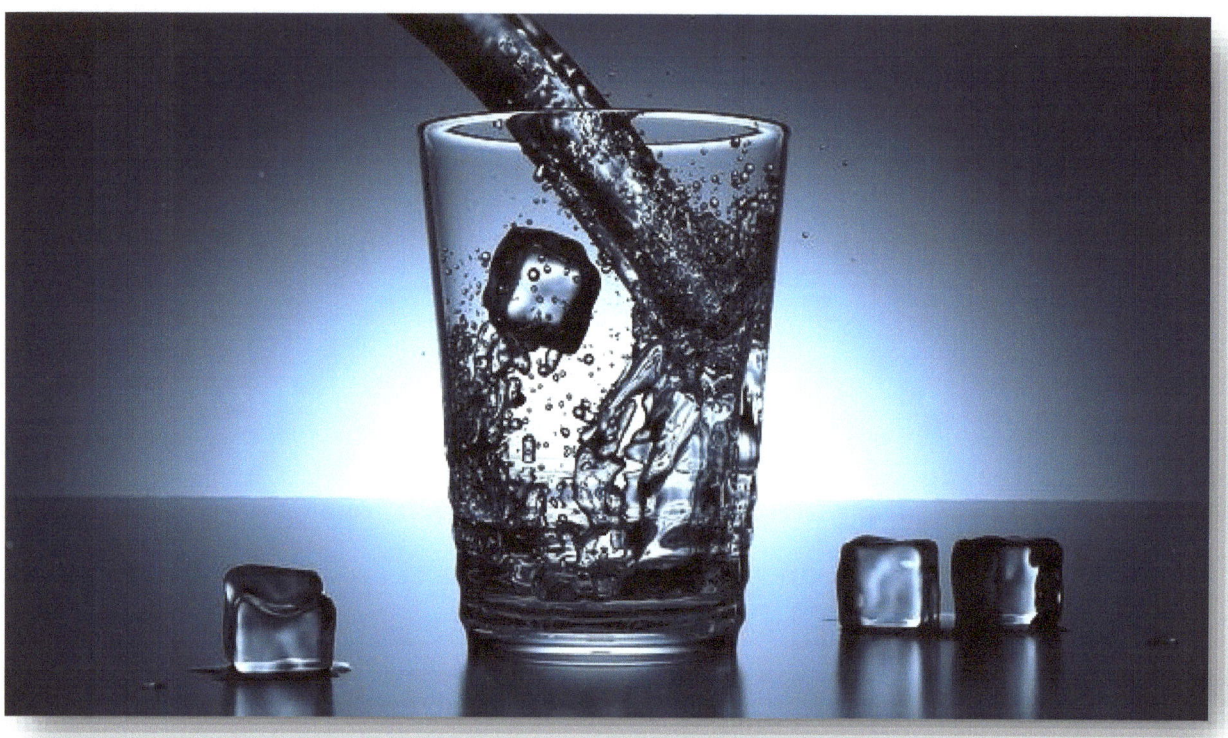

Hydration is a simple way to assist in relieving and overcoming gout. Drink enough water to keep the body hydrated and this will help dilute uric acid levels and help flush them out of the body through the urine.

This doesn't mean drinking beer or coffee, and if you smoke, it would be wise to give that up too. These vices contain substances that can increase the production of uric acid in the blood.

Exercise

Exercise can prevent future gout attacks by normalizing insulin levels that in turn normalize blood uric acid levels. Exercise also improves circulation and increases a healthy supply of blood to the joints.

Hot and Cold Therapy

If you have a gout attack, place an ice pack over the affected area for a couple of minutes. The coldness will numb the senses and ease the pain for a while. Usually when inflammation is a problem, cold is the answer for reducing swelling.

However, some patients prefer the soothing warmth instead. If this is you, try placing a hot towel over the affected area.

Whichever method is more effective depends on the affected person.

Conclusion

Gout is one of those conditions that can be prevented through a healthy diet and lifestyle. It can be easily managed and relieved without relying on synthetic medications for the rest of your life.

Knowing what food to eat and more importantly, what not to eat, to prevent gout is the key to managing and preventing gout attacks forever.

As the saying goes, "Prevention is always better than cure!"

Natural Pain Management

Regardless of which type of arthritis you are dealing with, you can very likely make changes to your diet and lifestyle to help with your arthritis pain management.

Making some dietary changes can significantly help reduce your inflammation. Incorporating more fish oils in your diet, staying hydrated and avoiding trigger foods can really make a difference to your pain levels.

Gluten-Free Diet

Many people find that once they adopt a gluten-free diet, they additionally become more limber. You can still enjoy your favorite carbohydrates such as breads and pastas; however, they just cannot be made from wheat, rye or barley.

Rice flour and coconut flour can be some great alternative options.

Physiotherapy

Many patients report an increase in mobility by working with a trained professional. Incorporating some specific exercises into your day can help you become more flexible over time. It is essential to move the joints in order to increase blood flow. Our blood nourishes muscle and bone tissue and over time can help stiff and stagnant joints feel less painful.

[Yoga](#) and Tai Chi

These two forms of exercise are excellent for gently stimulating your circulation and help 'wake up' stiff joints that have not been mobile or flexible for quite some time.

These two forms of exercise can be done at your own pace and within a short amount of time. You will soon notice how you can reach further and hold poses for longer.

It is vital to breathe deeply during your routines in order to help bring oxygenated blood to the joints, helping to facilitate the healing process.

Don't underestimate the healing powers of these two therapies. If you think of these types of therapies as being for the 'alternative lifestyle' people, perhaps you might like to take a better look and reconsider. Your arthritis pain may reduce greatly if you do.

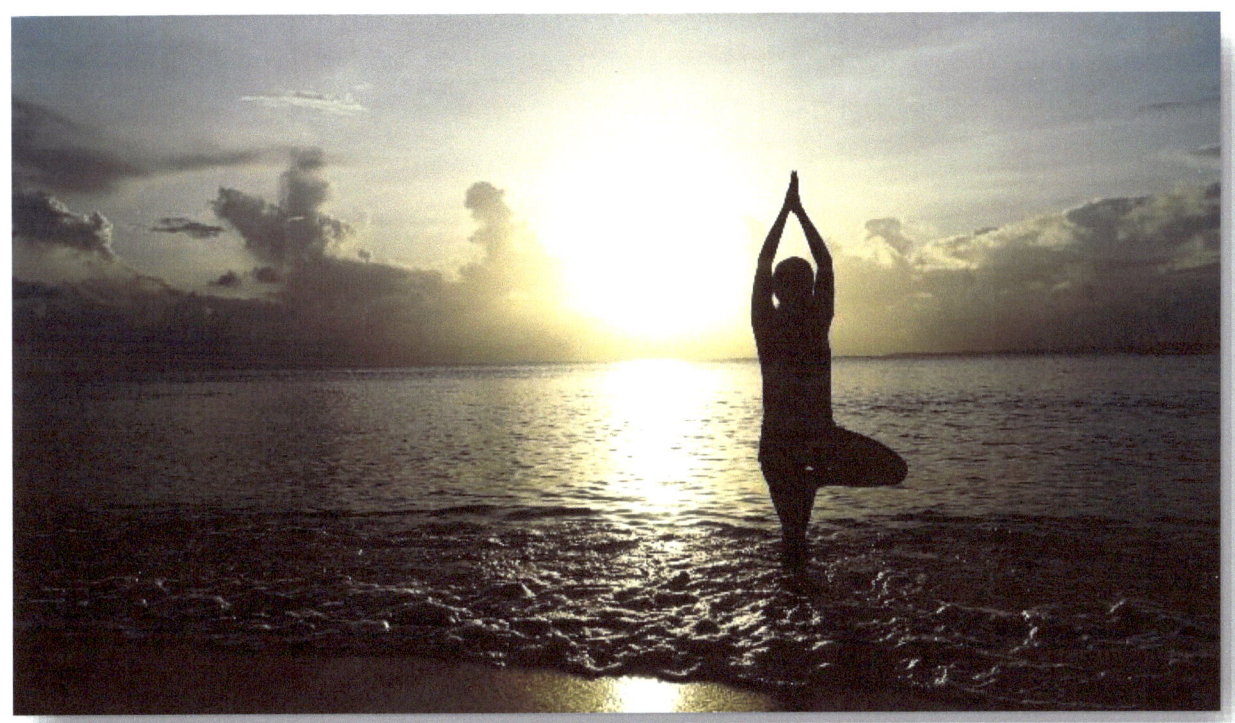

Anti-Inflammatory Herbs

Herbs are so multipurpose. Brewing some tea in the morning and before bed, adding some to the bath water in a homemade nylon bag or topically applying a compress on affected areas can make a positive difference. Most of the herbs used for reducing inflammation are very common and available.

Some of the best known anti-inflammatory herbs include:

- Turmeric or Curcuma longa
- Guaiacum or Lignum vitae
- Cowslip
- Yellow Dock

- German and Roman Chamomile
- Feverfew
- Fennel
- Devil's Claw and Mistletoe.

Aspirin-like Herbs

Many of the pain reliever medications available today originated from natural plants. Willow Bark for example, Wintergreen, Birch, White Poplar bark and Meadowsweet have been used since ancient times for alleviating pain. These are all natural herbs that are known to be similar to aspirin for reducing pain and inflammation.

Oily Fish

People take fish oils to improve their skin and help lubricate their joints. They are great for heart health and improving circulation, and can of course be beneficial for joint problems.

Great fish choices include cod, mackerel and herring. It is advised you include these in your meal plan, and eat at least two fish meals per week.

In countries such as Greenland, where oily fish is a regular part of the diet, heart disease is practically unheard of. What does that tell you?

Compresses

Another simple method for alleviating arthritis pain is to alternate hot and cold compresses to encourage blood flow to the affected area. Hot and cold therapy works by stimulating your own body's healing force.

Heat therapy provides pain relief by altering the sensation of pain as it stimulates blood circulation, while also dilating the blood vessels to reduce muscle spasms.

You may use heating pads, heat lamps, warm baths, or heated wash cloths for this kind of therapy.

Conversely, you may also reduce the swelling of your joints by using cold packs which help constrict your blood vessels. Although cold packs can be uncomfortable in the beginning, it helps numb pain and reduce inflammation, which in turn brings relief.

Weight Loss

Weight loss is one of the best ways to lessen the pain brought about by arthritis. Every pound you lose means less strain and pain on your joints. Some people experience complete relief from arthritis pain after losing 10 to 20 pounds.

A study revealed that losing 10% of bodyfat can significantly lessen arthritis pain and reduce inflammation.

Whatever your choice or choices, measures are available to so you can take some control and manage arthritic pain effectively.

Herbal Remedies for Natural Treatment

Many people find conventional anti-inflammatory medicines and aspirin or ibuprofen-based pain relievers hard to take on a regular basis. Some of these traditional remedies irritate people's stomachs when taken daily. Other arthritis sufferers simply prefer a more natural approach.

Incorporating the following herbal remedies into your current care routine may be beneficial. Remember to check with your health care provider prior to starting any new treatments.

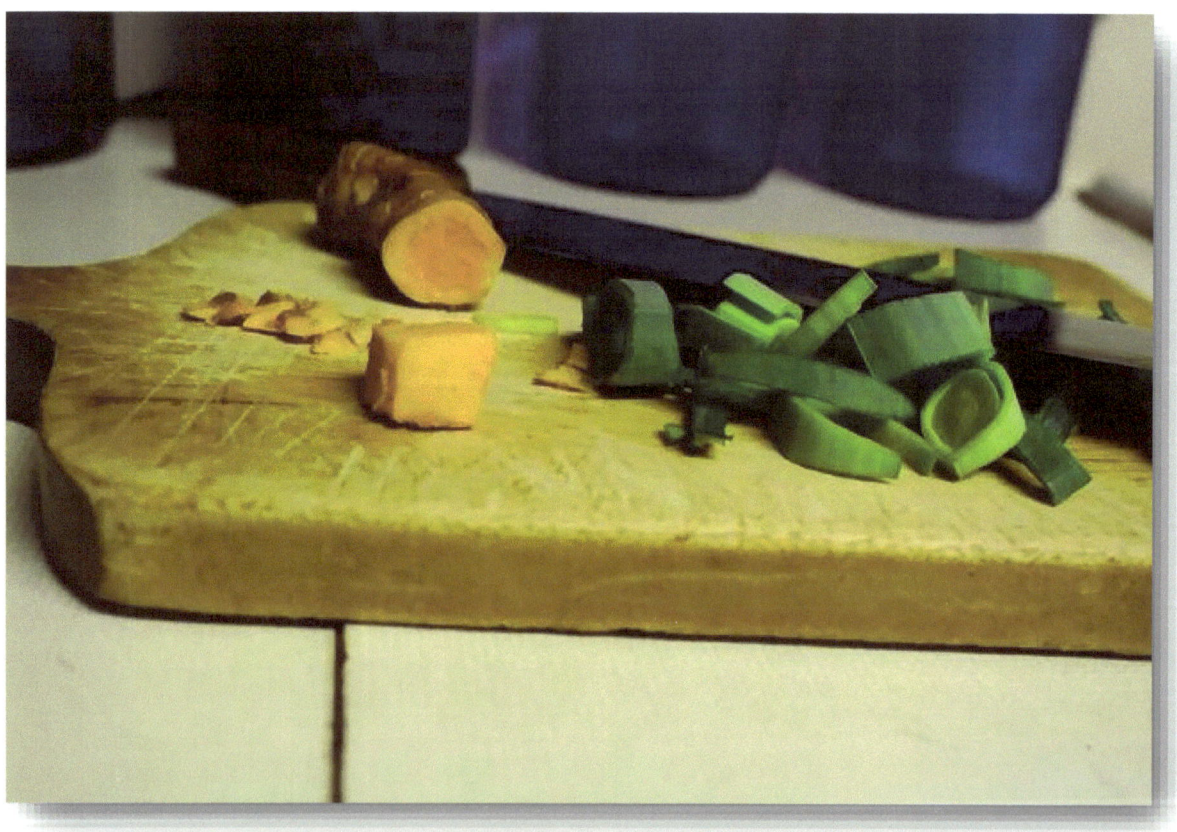

Two Popular Herbs for Arthritis Pain Relief

There are many herbs used to fight arthritis pain and inflammation. Here are two of the popular ones:

Turmeric

This yellow herb contains an active compound called curcumin which is known to work better than many traditional drugs used for giving arthritis relief.

Curcumin has potent anti-arthritic and anti-inflammatory properties. A research study revealed that participants who used curcumin were found to have a higher percentage of improvement of their symptoms than those individuals who were given the drug Voltaren.

The acting participants in the curcumin group withdrew from the study with no adverse effects. This was the first study conducted which set out to prove the safety and potency of curcumin for giving relief to arthritis sufferers.

Burdock Root

This herb is rich in fatty oils which have an anti-inflammatory effect. You can eat stir-fried burdock root, which is common in Asian cuisine.

You can also chop the fresh roots and add them to boiling water, then allow to steep for no more than ten minutes. Strain, then drink. If you do not have fresh burdock roots, you can also use dried roots.

Here are a few more herbal remedies for specific types of arthritis.

Psoriatic Arthritis

Helpful Teas

- 1 heaped teaspoon per cup of boiling water; Chickweed, Red Clover Flowers or Gotu Kola.
- Can be used in combination or as a single tea
- Allow to steep for 5 to 10 minutes.
- Dose is 1 cup, three times a day.

Topical

- Try massaging Evening Primrose oil, Jojoba oil or Mullein oil on the affected areas.
- A poultice made of Comfrey can be very soothing.
- Chickweed cream is additionally beneficial.

Liquid Extract

- Mix together equal parts of Gotu Kola, Echinacea and Devil's Claw.
- Dose is 30 to 60 drops three times a day prior to meals.

Additional Beneficial Herbs and Supplements

- Burdock, Thuja, Prickly Ash Bark, Boneset, Sarsaparilla, Fennel, Cod Liver Oil, Zinc, Magnesium, Sulphur, B-Complex, Vitamins A, C, D and E.

Osteoarthritis

Helpful Teas

- Comfrey Tea
- Celery Seed Tea made from 1 teaspoon of celery seeds to each cup of boiling water.
- Allow to steep for 15 minutes.
- Dose is half to 1 cup, three times a day, prior to meals.

Liquid Extract

- Mix together ¼ Tincture of Capsicum, 1 part Fennel, 1 part Devil's Claw, 1 part Bogbean and 2 parts White Willow.
- Dose is 1 teaspoon three times a day, in Nettle tea or water.

Additional Beneficial Herbs and Supplements

- Meadowsweet and Black Cohosh are natural sources of salicylic acid.
- Hawthorn is excellent for blood circulation.
- Inflammation of connective tissue can benefit greatly from Asafoetida.
- Yucca leaves, Guaiacum, Bladderwrack, and Devil's Claw.

Topical

- Capsicum cream and Jojoba oil rubbed onto affected areas.

Complementary Therapy

- Physiotherapy is helpful for increasing mobility.
- Alternate between hot and cold packs on affected joints twice a day.
- Epsom salt baths are soothing and recommended to be taken twice a week.

Rheumatoid Arthritis

Helpful Teas

- Mix together equal parts of Nettles, Bogbean and Alfalfa; 1 heaped teaspoon to each cup of boiling water
- Allow to steep for 5 to 10 minutes.
- Dose is 1 cup, three times a day.

Liquid Extract

- Mix together ½ Liquorice, ½ Wild Yam, 2 parts White Willow bark and ¼ Guaiacum.
- Dose is 1 to 2 teaspoons, three times a day.

Topical

- Wintergreen Lotion
- Evening Primrose oil
- Comfrey Poultice
- Hot fomentations (or poultice) of Chamomile, Ragwort or Hops.
- Any of the following aromatherapy massage oils - Rosemary, Pine, Cajeput or Juniper - mix 6 drops into 2 teaspoons of Almond oil and massage into stiff areas.

Additional Beneficial Herbs and Supplements

- Korean Ginseng, Siberian Ginseng, Devil's Claw, Balmony, Agrimony, Angelica Root, Cramp Bark, Prickly Ash Bark, White Willow Bark.

- Black Cohosh is especially useful if sciatica and lower back pain are present.

Complementary Therapy

- Crushed ice or frozen peas applied to affected area for 10 minute intervals
- Hydrotherapy

Treat Osteoarthritis Naturally

Osteoarthritis typically effects people over 50 and is common in menopausal women. It is characterized by stiffness and pain within the joints. It often presents in the knees, hands, hips and spine. Eventually the cartilage between the joints becomes worn; hence the nickname of "wear and tear" arthritis.

Although common in mature women, it doesn't mean you have to continually suffer from its painful effects. There are natural solutions you can turn to which we'll cover in a moment.

The reason a person may begin to suffer with this type of arthritis is usually due to dietary issues. Calcium salts may accumulate within the joints, causing small crystals of calcium hydroxyapatite to form. In an attempt to correct the condition, the biochemical changes within the cartilage can cause hyperplasia, or an overgrowth of bone cells.

The elderly population commonly experiences a diminished supply of HCL or hydrochloric acid in their stomach. HCL is necessary for calcium metabolism to occur properly.

For individuals dealing with less stomach acid, incorporating 2 teaspoons of apple cider vinegar in a glass of water and sipping with each meal can significantly help.

Natural Arthritis Treatments

Warm, Dry Climate

Arthritis sufferers who live in coastal regions or areas with lots of humidity, often report more "aches and pains" as compared to those who live in a more arid climate. So, depending where you live, visit or move to a warm, less humid climate for relief from pain. It's not a remedy in a bottle, but it's a great remedy!

Topical Treatments

Try taking warm baths with Epsom salts twice a week. This is a great way to relax body and mind and absorb some magnesium through your skin.

Capsicum cream made from cayenne pepper is another excellent option for stimulating circulation and bringing blood flow to stagnant joints. It is easy to make your own using unscented lotion, coconut oil or olive oil. Break open a capsule and gradually increase the amount as your skin tolerates it.

Packs made from Jojoba oil are also very soothing. Cold and hot compresses twice a day on affected areas, followed by using a cold compress at bedtime can significantly reduce inflammation.

Diet

Sticking to a low sodium, high fiber diet is beneficial. Increasing your consumption of oily fish or taking fish oil supplements will help to lubricate your joints from the inside.

It is recommended to avoid citrus fruit and lemons. Drinking lemon juice in a glass of water may help to remove some of the calculi from the body and taste very refreshing; however, in excess, it can begin to take calcium out of the bones.

Cod Liver Oil

By the process of osmosis, this excellent iodized oil can nourish and reach the cartilage. It promotes an increase in elasticity. Taking 2 teaspoons once a day can be easily done if you mix with juice or add into a smoothie.

If you simply cannot stand the taste, try the capsules.

Supplements

Zinc 25mg, Vitamin E 400 iu, Vitamin A 7500 iu, Vitamin B6 25mg and Pantothenic acid 10mg have been successful. If you are taking a multivitamin, check how much of the above you are already taking each day.

It is wise to consult your family physician prior to taking any new vitamins, herbs or supplements, especially if you are taking prescription medication.

Reduce Arthritis Inflammation With Bromelain

According to the National Institute of Health, bromelain can be an effective treatment for arthritis as well as relieve other inflammation pain. It also reduces swelling and bruising, and hastens the healing process.

Bromelain is a combination of enzymes and compounds that can be extracted from a family of plant, Bromeliaceae, or more commonly known as the pineapple.

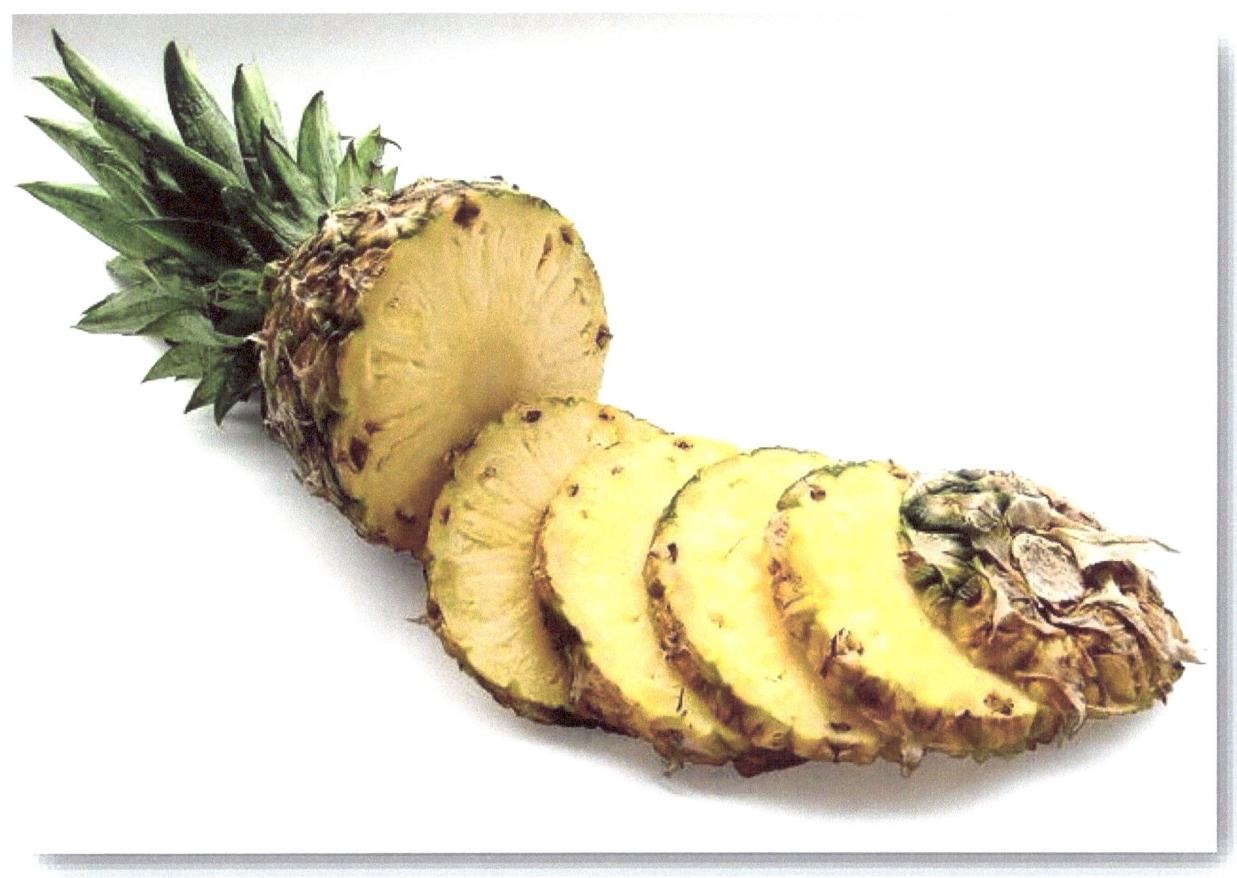

Bromelain is a digestive enzyme and known for supporting the digestive processes. It can cause slight stomach discomfort in some people, due to its powerful digestive enzymes.

It has many medicinal benefits and has been used throughout history. Today, if you look at some of the natural pain relieving supplements available, you may find bromelain is one of the major ingredients. That's because it helps fight inflammation pain and other body aches and pains.

You can purchase 'Bromelain Supplements', which quite often have a pineapple picture on them.

Bromelain has been shown to interfere with tumor growth. It is also a natural blood thinning agent. For this reason, anyone who is considering taking it should speak to their health care professional first.

This is especially important for anyone who is taking medication such as aspirin or Warfarin to prevent their blood clotting, as well as anyone likely to be undergoing surgery.

Bromelain for Osteoarthritis Pain

Bromelain can be taken as a natural supplement and this is the easiest way to obtain the enzyme in dosage amounts that can prove beneficial. In addition, taking bromelain with other herbs that contain trypsin and rutin has shown to be helpful in patients with osteoarthritis. Some proprietary natural remedies are available that have these ingredients combined in one product.

Studies have been done to test the efficacy of bromelain against arthritic pain, and the results showed that bromelain was just as effective as non-steroidal anti-inflammatory drugs used for arthritis treatment.

Other experiments included some participants given a placebo, and others bromelain. The participants given bromelain found their inflammation pain was reduced, whereas the placebo group had no improvement. This showed the efficacy of bromelain as a pain reliever and anti-inflammatory.

Lack of further experiments has not confirmed the efficacy of using bromelain against rheumatoid arthritis although it is very promising against osteoarthritis.

Bromelain – Natural Pain Reliever and Anti-Inflammatory

Bromelain has been used for treating not only arthritis, but also back pain and strains because it is an all-natural pain reliever, and doesn't have negative side-effects.

Experiments have also been conducted for pain relief and bruising. Results were proof enough that individuals who had taken bromelain healed faster and experienced less pain compared to others in the test who did not take bromelain.

The time taken to heal had reduced by almost half for those participants taking bromelain, compared to other participants who were prescribed medications and those who were given placebos.

Bromelain is an effective, natural alternative to anti-inflammatory prescription drugs. However, as stated earlier, always check with your physician before taking any natural supplements, especially if on any form of medication.

Inflammation-Causing Foods

Although we all tend to view inflammation negatively, inflammation serves as our body's way of responding to injury. It is during the inflammation process that the body's defense mechanism becomes active, in part by making sure that the immune cells are being sent to the affected area.

In addition to the immune cells being sent to the affected area, so too are key nutrients. These are both vital for the body to begin its repair and recovery functions.

While this can be a benefit in an acute or injury situation, when inflammation is sustained or chronic it can become more a part of the problem than the solution. There is increasing recognition that a large range of painful, debilitating and even dangerous health issues are related to chronic inflammation.

The foods we eat can cause, worsen or reduce inflammation. If you have a problem with arthritis, reducing inflammation will be one your goals. As part of your self-treatment, the foods listed below are ones you should try to avoid.

Trans Fats

Trans fats are commonly found in processed foods. As a wise consumer, you should take the time to read the labels and avoid those food products that contain partially hydrogenated oils, as they can exacerbate an inflammation problem.

Sugar

Sugar and simple carbohydrates cause a rapid rise in blood sugar levels. If you consume any type of sugar, such as sucrose, lactose, and high fructose corn syrup, this occurs. In response to the elevated blood sugar levels, the insulin levels go up correspondingly, which triggers the body's pro-inflammatory response.

If this is a common occurrence (and it usually is) the person will be likely to develop chronic inflammation issues.

Refined Grains

White bread and other foods which are made up of refined grains are fairly quickly broken down into sugar. Therefore, these fast-digesting caloric foods will contribute to an increase in inflammation.

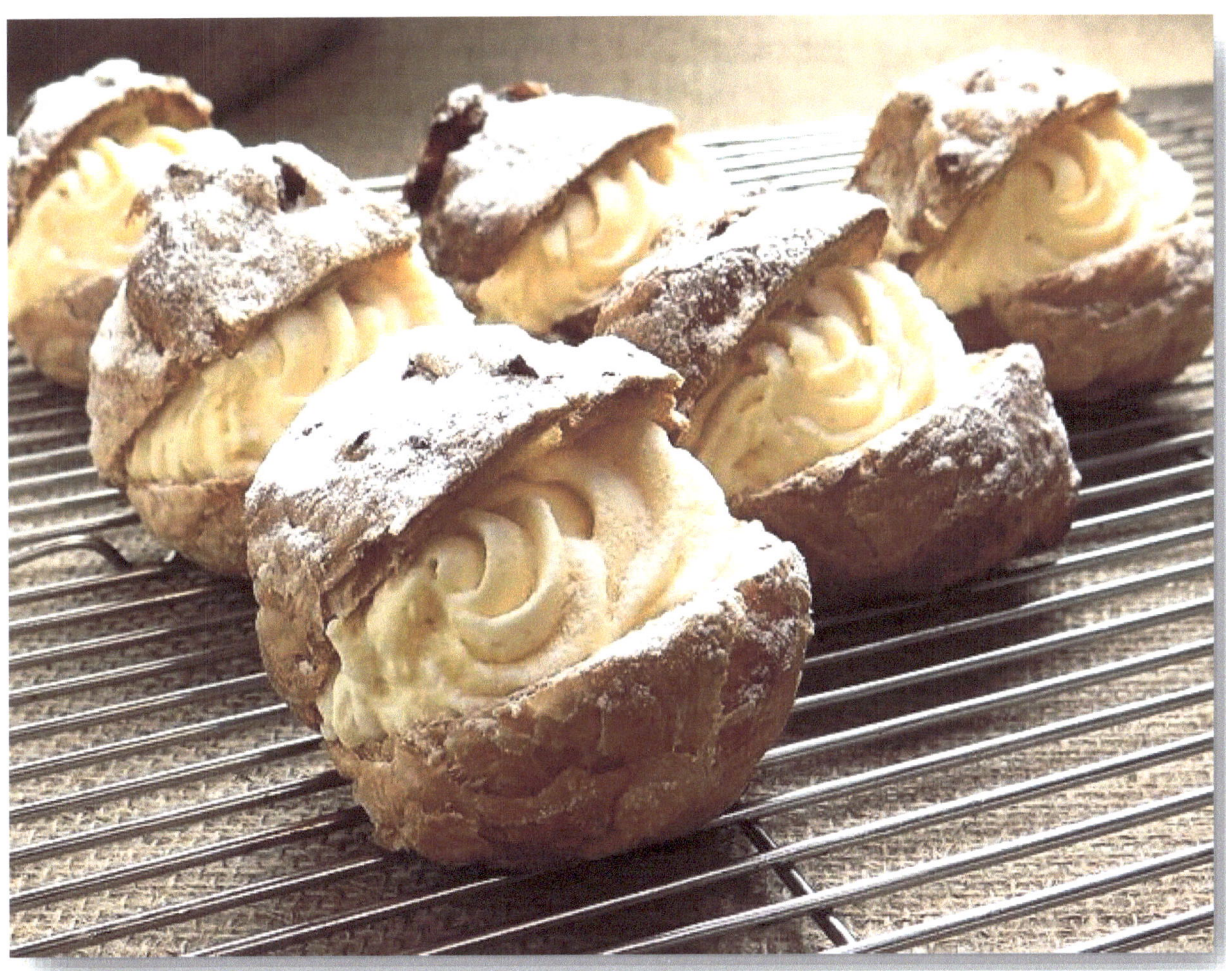

Dairy Foods

Dairy foods are getting blamed for many health problems today. Many people have excluded dairy as part of an elimination diet and found their health problems lessened. Some have found they only needed to abstain from milk, whereas others have had to forego all dairy products.

A person who is lactose intolerant (and they may not even know) may be consuming dairy products daily and not even realize they are exacerbating an inflammation problem with their dietary choices.

Even if you are not lactose intolerant, dairy products may still be adding to the collective inputs that are toxifying your system, which your body responds to with an inflammation response.

Be Your Own Food Tester

Read all food labels so you truly know what you are eating. Keep a food journal and see if you can see a recurring pattern. If so, take the steps to remove these types of foods from your diet and reduce your inflammation pain in the process.

By a combination of maintaining a food diary and selectively eliminating food types from their diet, many people have greatly reduced their painful symptoms that are caused by inflammation, as well as improving their overall health and wellness.

WHAT TO AVOID

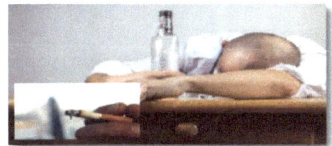   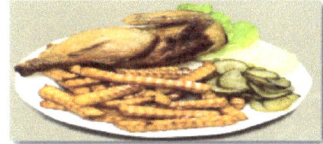

Alcohol & Tobacco

Those who smoke face a higher risk of developing rheumatoid arthritis while alcoholics are more at risk of having gout.

Stop smoking, reduce your alcohol intake and work towards having healthy lifestyle choices.

Fried and Processed Foods

Reduced intake of fried and processed foods helps reduce inflammation while restoring the body's natural defenses.

Incorporate more plant-based foods in your daily diet.

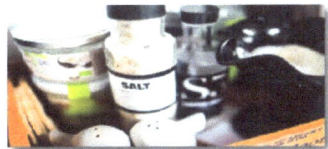   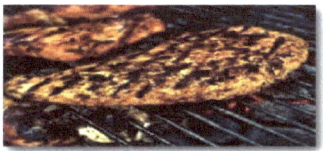

Salt & Preservatives

Excess salt consumption causes inflammation. Salt is used in processed and preserved foods to extend their shelf life. Eating large amounts of these foods will result in more inflammation.

Reduce if not eliminate processed, preserved and microwavable foods to better manage your arthritis symptoms.

Beware of AGEs

Reduce consumption of foods cooked at high temperatures such as roasting, grilling, frying and baking.

These can can contain toxins which are called Advanced Glycation End products or AGEs.

These AGEs damage the body's proteins, causing inflammation that leads to the development of conditions such as arthritis.

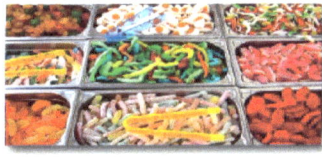   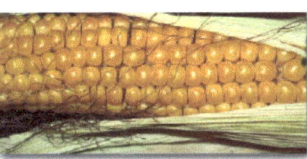

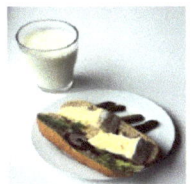

Sugars & Refined Carbs

As much as possible, eliminate sugar and simple carbohydrates from your diet.

These 'foods' have little nutrient value but promote painful inflammation.

Corn Oil

Baked goods contain high amounts of omega 6 fatty acids which, in excess, can trigger inflammation.

Choose anti-inflammatory foods and those that contain omega 3 fatty acids such as flax seeds, olive oil, pumpkin seeds and nuts.

Dairy products

Dairy products contain protein that may exacerbate inflammation as it irritates the tissues surrounding the joints. Instead of sourcing your protein from animal-meat alone, eat more plant-based sources of protein such as quinoa, beans, lentils, nuts, spinach and tofu.

Inflammation-Reducing Foods

Just as eating certain foods can exacerbate inflamed problem areas, there are foods and food types that can be consumed that can help reduce inflammation.

Making healthy food choices for reducing inflammation is a great start to managing arthritic pain. It is also very empowering to take simple steps yourself that can improve your condition and reduce your pain and discomfort.

Here are a few foods you may like to add to your diet plan to help win the fight against inflammation.

Green Leafy Vegetables

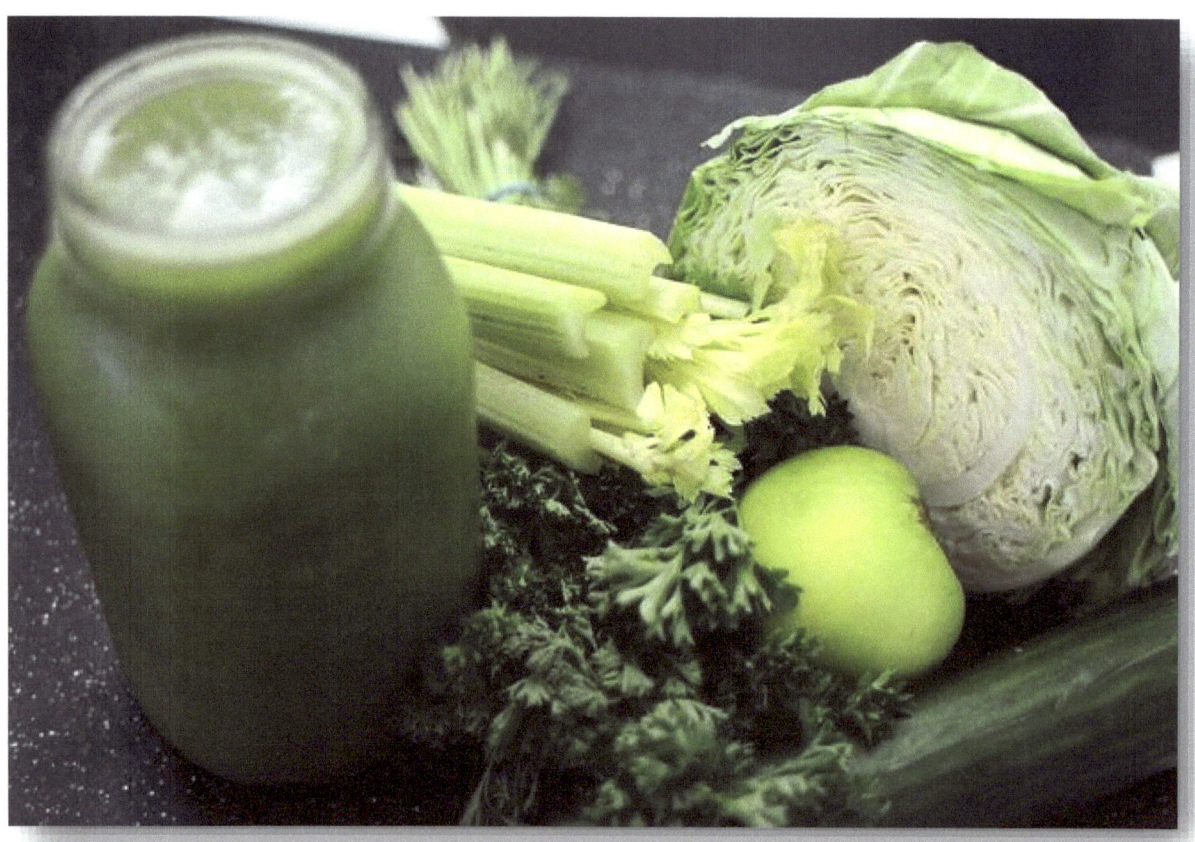

As always, 'green leafy vegetables' are foods you can easily add to your anti-inflammatory diet. There are many green vegetables to choose from, such as broccoli, bok choy, spinach etc.

If you don't like your greens or are sick of being told to eat them up, try having green vegetable smoothies instead!

Fatty Fish – For Omega 3 Fatty Acids

Salmon, tuna, mackerel and other fatty fish are rich sources of Omega-3 fatty acids that are beneficial for reducing inflammation. To achieve maximum benefit, cook your fish in a healthy manner. Avoid fried and salted fish. Instead, opt for baked, boiled or steamed fish, and try not to overcook.

If you can eat fatty fish on a regular basis you will boost your health massively! Fresh fish is always better than taking fish oils supplements, however, if you can't get enough in your diet, it is still very beneficial to supplement when necessary.

Kelp – 'Fucoidan'

Kelp is a good source of the anti-inflammatory compound known as fucoidan. Fucoidan is a complex carbohydrate and acts as an anti-inflammatory agent.

Fucoidan has other benefits too. It is beneficial for collagen synthesis and its fiber content promotes a feeling of fullness. It also helps lower the speed of fat absorption. Both these benefits are appreciated by those looking to lose weight.

Other rich sources of fucoidan include wakame, kombu and arame.

Turmeric

Studies have shown that turmeric beats even ginger when it comes to fighting inflammation and arthritis. You may also try curcumin, which is the most active compound of turmeric.

Cacao – Nature's Chocolate

The Journal of Cardiovascular Pharmacology reveals that cacao helps fight inflammation because it has the ability to decrease the levels of inflammatory chemicals found in the body. Just make sure to choose the dark chocolate.

Red Grapes

Red grapes contain resveratrol which helps lower levels of inflammation by controlling nitric oxide levels, which can be responsible for cellular damage and inflammation.

Apples

Indeed, an apple a day keeps inflammation at bay. The Journal of Neuroscience reveals that an apple has the ability to suppress inflammation proteins because of its quercetin content. Pineapples and blueberries also contain quercetin.

Pineapples additionally contain an enzyme, known as bromelain, another anti-inflammatory fighter.

Celery

Celery has become extremely popular in helping with arthritis and inflammation. Many supplements made with celery seeds are available for this purpose. Celery is an easy food to keep fresh in your fridge for nibbling on daily.

From the list above, add as many as you can to your next grocery list. Chronic inflammation doesn't have to be accepted as unavoidable in your life, however the onus is on you to take action to overcome it.

Any time you are able to this by employing diet and lifestyle factors, rather than simply taking "medicine" you will be doing your health a huge favor.

FOODS TO EAT

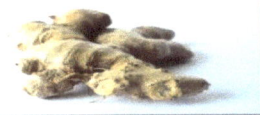   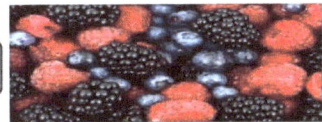

Ginger

The Journal of Medicinal Food provides proof that ginger plays a role in providing relief to people who are plagued with arthritis.

To incorporate more ginger into your diet, try adding grated fresh ginger to your sautéed veggies, tea and into some of your baked goods.

Anthocyanins

Increased intake of foods that contain these antioxidants will help reduce inflammation caused by rheumatoid arthritis.

These antioxidants can be obtained from strawberries, raspberries, grapes and blackberries.

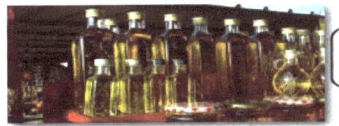   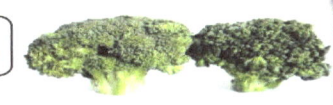

Olive oil

This oil helps reduce pain by preventing stiffness of the areas affected with arthritis. Its anti-inflammatory effects can be attributed to its oleic acid content that acts as antioxidants.

To ensure that you get enough olive oil each day, stop buying ready-made salad dressings and prepare your own.

Broccoli

Broccoli and other cruciferous veggies help prevent the onset of arthritis.

Besides broccoli, you may also include kale, bok choy, cauliflower, cabbage and Brussel sprouts to your diet.

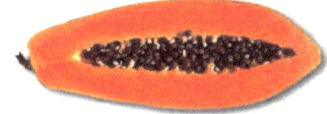   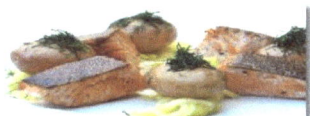

Beta-cryptoxanthin

These antioxidants, which are helpful for the prevention of arthritis will be converted into vitamin A once ingested in the body.

Make sure that your daily diet includes foods that are rich in beta-cryptoxanthin such as pumpkins, squash, tangerines, sweet peppers, collard greens and papayas.

Omega-3 fats

A reduced intake of foods that are high in omega 6 and increased consumption of omega 3 fats helps reduce the production of inflammation-causing enzymes.

Eat more flaxseeds, walnut, sardines, mackerel and salmon and avoid if not reduce intake of fast foods, meat, sunflower oil and junk foods.

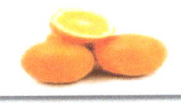   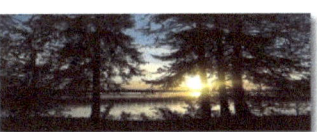

Vitamin C

Studies show that increased intake of foods that are rich in vitamin C will help reduce the risk of developing rheumatoid arthritis.

Do not rely solely on supplements for your daily dose of vitamin C. Eat foods that are also good sources of this nutrient such as fresh fruits and vegetables.

Vitamin D

People who have enough vitamin D in their bodies are less likely to develop arthritis according to a study which had 29,000 women as participants.

Aim for at least 20 minutes a day exposure to early morning sunlight which serves as the best source of vitamin D.

Conclusion

There is no one arthritis, or one cure. Some types of arthritis are considered incurable at this point in time, however information and support exists to help in managing the symptoms and effects, to provide the best life experience possible in spite of the condition.

Some types of arthritis fall into the lifestyle disease category. While it can be disconcerting to realize that your own actions or inactions may have contributed to your condition, it also means you have the option to make changes that can also positively affect your life.

If you are so affected, instead of basing your arthritis management on pain-killers, it may be time to make the changes to diet and exercise that can help the symptoms stay away for good.

Let me share a story with you on my experience with prescription medication that was prescribed to reduce the joint pain from my osteoarthritis. I have osteoarthritis in my shoulders, wrists and hands. I was taking diclofenac prescribed by my doctor for the pain. And while it did help with the pain, unbeknownst to me it was interfering with the functioning of my kidneys. I didn't find that out until I went in for a hernia operation and the anesthesiologist mentioned that my kidney values were much higher than they should be for someone my age and in good shape.

He asked what medications I was taking and when I mentioned diclofenac, he said that was the one causing the problem and that I should stop taking it and see if my doctor would prescribe something else. In the end, I stopped taking it and did not get a replacement. My kidney values were recently checked again a year later and have since returned to normal. I can live with joint pain, but I can't live well without functioning kidneys.

What I have found now that works the best for me is exercise – one hour three times per week and eating an inflammation reducing diet. And while I do have some pain on cold damp days, most days it is tolerable. This was a case where the side effects from the medication were worse than the condition it was treating.

Recommended Resource

The Beginner's Guide to Joint Health is the ultimate guide for understanding the most common health dilemma that affected millions of people — joint problems.

What you are about to discover in this guide is everything you need to know about joint health. Plus, scientifically proven methods for relieving and reducing the effect of joint pain.

If you are suffering from aches, pains, and creaky joints, or you just want to take effective measures to avoid this problem... then this guide is definitely for you.

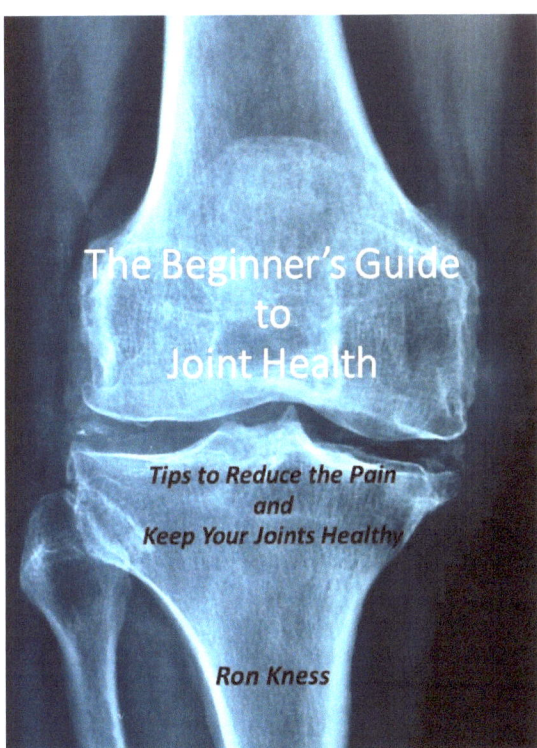

Here Are The Things You Will Discover In The Beginner's Guide to Joint Health:

- 3 things you don't want to happen when you don't take care of your joints

- How to know if your joints are damaged. (Here are 4 signs to look for!)

- Symptoms of the 5 common joint problems you must know

- If you find it hard to climb the stairs or to bend down... read Chapter 2 immediately.

- The ONE thing you can do to prevent joint damage & improve joint strengths

- 4 specific joint exercises you can do to strengthen your joints

- 3 key things to keep in mind when performing joint exercises

- The TWO most important nutrients for joint health (Revealed in Chapter 4)

- One of the best food to eat when you have inflammation

- 6 types of food (and drinks) to avoid when you have joint problems

- How your body weight affects your joints (and what to do about it.)

- How to do a simple 'standing' posture exercise that will reduce the stress on your knees, legs, and back

- 9 simple home remedies to relieve joint aches (This is for people who want to avoid the side effects of prescribed drugs!)

- 7 must-have supplements backed by scientific research for optimum joint health

- One common mistake thing most people ignored that 'secretly' degrades their joint health without them knowing!

- 4 treatments to relieve excruciating joint aches!

This is the Golden Key for those who want to:

- Reduce the pain associated with joints

- Reverse arthritis and other common joint problems

- Avoid taking over-the-counter medications by opting for simple home remedies

- Move freely without experiencing any sorts of pain

- Restore their youthful mobility & flexibility

- Lead a healthier & happier life

Get your copy today and keep your joints healthy and reduce the pain!

Referenced Books

[Osteoarthritis: Control It or It Will Control You](https://www.amazon.com/gp/product/153352159X) - https://www.amazon.com/gp/product/153352159X

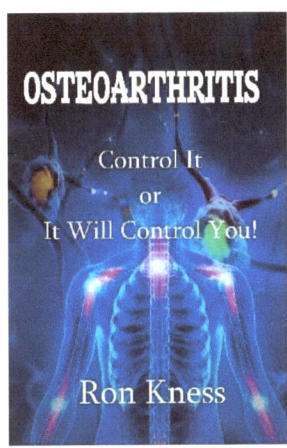

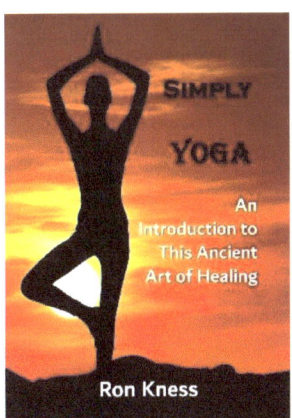

[Simply Yoga](https://www.amazon.com/Simply-Yoga-Introduction-Ancient-Healing/dp/1720135355) - https://www.amazon.com/Simply-Yoga-Introduction-Ancient-Healing/dp/1720135355

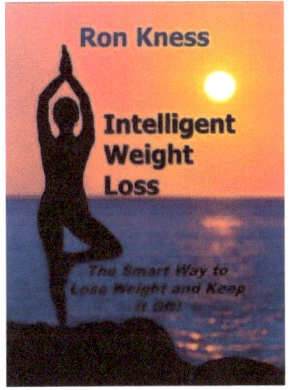

[Intelligent Weight Loss](https://www.amazon.com/gp/product/1718645724) - https://www.amazon.com/gp/product/1718645724

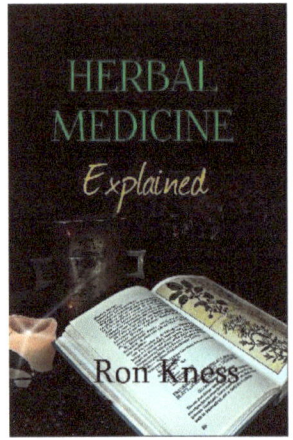

Herbal Medicine Explained - https://www.amazon.com/Herbal-Medicine-Explained-Healing-Natural/dp/1545079315

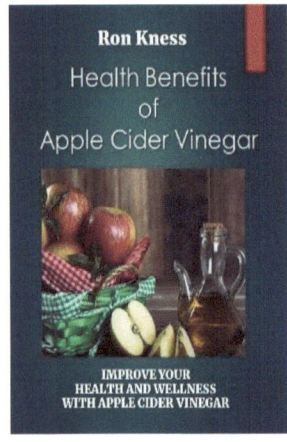

Health Benefits of Apple Cider Vinegar - https://www.amazon.com/gp/product/1790396026

About the Author

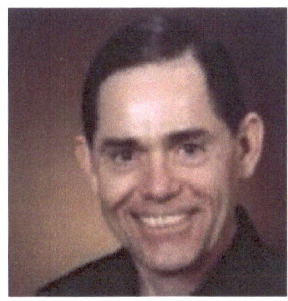

I have published numerous books on Amazon (both for Kindle and in paperback), along with other publishing platforms.

While most of my books are on health and fitness in general, I also write on baby boomer and older citizen health issues and have a recent interest in creating and printing journals/ planners and other printable products. A complete list of our published products on Amazon can be found at https://www.amazon.com/Ron-Kness/e/B0072M6PYO.

Besides my own writing, I also ghostwrite ebooks, books, reports, articles, blogs and do Kindle conversions for clients on a variety of topics. Contact me at Ron Kness Writing for a quote.

Today my wife and I are retired from our careers and live in San Tan Valley, AZ. I now write as a retirement business where you'll find me happily sitting in my office typing away on my laptop as I work on my next book or ghostwriting project . . . that is if we are not traveling on a cruise ship - our new-found mode of travel.